DR. BARBARA QUICK AND EASY 7-DAYS JUICE DETOX

Uncover holistic and herbal remedies to cleanse and detox your whole body, skin, kidney, liver, lungs for optimal health

Ben Hans

Table of Contents

COPYRIGHT © 2023

CHAPTER ONE

Introduction to Dr. Barbara's Herbal Juice Detox Program

Dr. Barbara's Herbal Juice Detox Program is a comprehensive approach to cleansing and rejuvenating the body using natural ingredients and herbal formulations. Developed by Dr. Barbara, a renowned holistic health practitioner, this program aims to promote detoxification, weight loss, improved digestion, and overall well-being.

Understanding Detoxification

Detoxification is the process of eliminating toxins and waste products from the body to improve health and vitality. Our bodies are exposed to various toxins from the environment, such as air pollution, pesticides in food, and chemicals in personal care products. Additionally, poor dietary choices, stress, and sedentary lifestyles can further burden our bodies with toxins.

The liver, kidneys, skin, lungs, and lymphatic system are the primary organs involved in detoxification. These organs work together to neutralize and eliminate toxins through processes such as sweating, urination, and bowel movements. However, when the body is overwhelmed with toxins or when these organs are not functioning optimally, detoxification may become inefficient, leading to symptoms such as fatigue, digestive issues, and skin problems.

The Importance of Herbal Medicine in Detoxification

Herbal medicine has been used for centuries in various cultures as a natural way to support detoxification and promote overall health. Herbs contain bioactive compounds that have been shown to have antioxidant, anti-inflammatory, and detoxifying properties. These compounds help support the body's natural detoxification processes and may enhance the function of the liver, kidneys, and other detox organs.

Dr. Barbara's Herbal Juice Detox Program incorporates a variety of medicinal herbs known for their detoxifying properties. These herbs are carefully selected and formulated to synergistically support detoxification, improve digestion, boost energy levels, and promote overall wellness.

Key Components of Dr. Barbara's Herbal Juice Detox Program

1. **Herbal Juice Blends**: The cornerstone of Dr. Barbara's program is the herbal juice blends, which are specially formulated to support detoxification and nourish the body with essential nutrients. These juices are made from organic fruits, vegetables, and medicinal herbs known for their

detoxifying properties. Each blend is designed to target specific detox organs and promote overall cleansing and rejuvenation.

2. **Herbal Supplements**: In addition to the herbal juice blends, Dr. Barbara's program may include herbal supplements to further support detoxification and address specific health concerns. These supplements may contain herbs such as milk thistle, dandelion root, and turmeric, which are known for their liver-protective and detoxifying effects.

3. **Nutritional Guidance**: Proper nutrition is essential for supporting detoxification and maintaining overall health. Dr. Barbara's program includes personalized nutritional guidance to help participants make healthy dietary choices during the detox process and beyond. This may involve recommendations for whole foods, organic produce, and specific dietary modifications to support detoxification and optimize health.

4. **Lifestyle Recommendations**: In addition to dietary changes, Dr. Barbara's program may include lifestyle recommendations to enhance the detoxification process and promote overall well-being. This may involve practices such as stress management techniques, regular exercise, adequate sleep, and mindfulness practices to support holistic health and vitality.

5. **Educational Resources**: Education is a key component of Dr. Barbara's Herbal Juice Detox Program. Participants receive comprehensive educational resources, including articles, videos, and guides, to help them understand the detox process, learn about the benefits of herbal medicine, and make informed choices about their health and wellness.

Benefits of Dr. Barbara's Herbal Juice Detox Program

1. **Detoxification**: By supporting the body's natural detoxification processes, Dr. Barbara's program helps eliminate toxins and waste products, leaving participants feeling lighter, more energized, and rejuvenated.

2. **Weight Loss**: Many participants experience weight loss as a result of the detox process, as excess toxins stored in fat cells are released and eliminated from the body. Additionally, the program promotes healthy eating habits and lifestyle changes that can support long-term weight management.

3. **Improved Digestion**: The herbal juice blends and dietary recommendations in Dr. Barbara's program can help improve digestion and alleviate symptoms such as bloating, gas, and constipation. By supporting gut health and promoting the elimination of toxins, participants may experience better digestion and overall digestive wellness.

4. **Increased Energy Levels**: Detoxification can help remove obstacles to energy flow in the body, leading to increased vitality and energy levels. Many participants report feeling more energetic and focused after completing Dr. Barbara's program.

5. **Enhanced Well-being**: By promoting detoxification, healthy eating habits, and lifestyle changes, Dr. Barbara's program can enhance overall well-being and quality of life. Participants may experience improvements in mood, sleep, skin health, and mental clarity, leading to a greater sense of vitality and vitality.

In conclusion, Dr. Barbara's Herbal Juice Detox Program offers a comprehensive and holistic approach to cleansing and rejuvenating the body using natural ingredients and herbal formulations. By supporting detoxification, weight loss, improved digestion, and overall well-being, this program empowers participants to take control of their health and embark on a journey towards optimal wellness.

CHAPTER TWO
Understanding the Benefits of Herbal Juice Detoxification

Herbal juice detoxification has gained popularity as a natural and effective way to cleanse the body, promote health, and rejuvenate from within. In this comprehensive exploration, we delve into the myriad benefits of herbal juice detoxification, understanding its impact on various aspects of health and well-being.

Detoxification and Cleansing

Detoxification is the process of eliminating harmful toxins and waste products from the body. Our modern lifestyles expose us to numerous toxins from environmental pollutants, processed foods, and stress, which can accumulate in the body over time and lead to various health issues. Herbal juice detoxification aids the body's natural detoxification processes, supporting organs such as the liver, kidneys, and digestive system in flushing out toxins. Herbal juices are rich in antioxidants, vitamins, minerals, and phytonutrients that help neutralize and eliminate toxins, promoting overall cleansing and rejuvenation.

Weight Loss and Metabolic Support

Herbal juice detoxification is often associated with weight loss, as it helps to eliminate excess toxins stored in fat cells. By cleansing the digestive system and improving metabolic function, herbal juices can enhance the body's ability to burn fat and maintain a healthy weight. Additionally, many herbal ingredients have thermogenic properties, which can increase metabolism and promote fat loss. Incorporating herbal juices into a balanced diet and lifestyle can support sustainable weight management and improve body composition.

Improved Digestion and Gut Health

The digestive system plays a crucial role in overall health, and herbal juice detoxification can help optimize its function. Herbal juices are often rich in fiber, enzymes, and prebiotics, which support digestion and promote the growth of beneficial gut bacteria. By cleansing the digestive tract and removing accumulated waste, herbal juices can alleviate symptoms such as bloating, gas, and constipation, leading to improved digestive health and regularity. Additionally, certain herbs, such as ginger and peppermint, have been traditionally used to soothe digestive discomfort and promote gastrointestinal motility.

Boosted Energy and Vitality

Toxins and waste products can impair energy production and circulation in the body, leading to fatigue and sluggishness. Herbal juice detoxification helps remove these obstacles to energy flow, allowing the body to function more efficiently and effectively. The vitamins, minerals, and antioxidants found in herbal juices nourish the body at a cellular level, supporting optimal energy production and vitality. Many participants report feeling more energized, focused, and mentally clear after completing a herbal juice detox program, experiencing a renewed sense of vitality and well-being.

Enhanced Immune Function

The immune system plays a critical role in defending the body against infections and diseases, and herbal juice detoxification can help support its function. By reducing the burden of toxins and oxidative stress, herbal juices support immune system health and resilience. Many herbs used in detoxification blends, such as echinacea, astragalus, and elderberry, have immune-boosting properties that help strengthen the body's natural defenses. By promoting overall health and vitality, herbal juice detoxification can enhance immune function and reduce the risk of illness.

Reduced Inflammation and Oxidative Stress

Chronic inflammation and oxidative stress are underlying factors in many chronic diseases, including heart disease, diabetes, and autoimmune conditions. Herbal juice detoxification helps reduce inflammation and oxidative stress by providing the body with a rich source of antioxidants and anti-inflammatory compounds. Ingredients such as turmeric, green tea, and berries have been shown to have potent anti-inflammatory and antioxidant properties, helping protect cells from damage and promoting overall health and longevity.

Balanced Hormones and Improved Skin Health

Hormonal imbalances and skin issues are common concerns that can be addressed through herbal juice detoxification. Many herbs used in detoxification blends, such as dandelion root, burdock root, and milk thistle, support hormonal balance by promoting liver health and detoxification. By clearing excess hormones and toxins from the body, herbal juices can help alleviate symptoms such as acne, PMS, and hormonal fluctuations. Additionally, the vitamins, minerals, and antioxidants found in herbal juices support skin health from the inside out, promoting a clear, radiant complexion.

Stress Reduction and Mental Clarity

Detoxification is not only beneficial for the body but also for the mind. Herbal juice detoxification can help reduce stress and promote mental clarity by supporting the body's natural stress response systems. Ingredients such as adaptogenic herbs (e.g., ashwagandha, rhodiola) help modulate the body's response to stress, promoting a sense of calm and relaxation. Many participants report feeling more mentally clear, focused, and emotionally balanced after completing a herbal juice detox program, experiencing enhanced cognitive function and overall well-being.

In conclusion, herbal juice detoxification offers a wide range of benefits for overall health and well-being, including detoxification and cleansing, weight loss and metabolic support, improved digestion and gut health, boosted energy and vitality, enhanced immune function, reduced inflammation and oxidative stress, balanced hormones and improved skin health, and stress reduction and mental clarity. By incorporating herbal juices into a balanced diet and lifestyle, individuals can support their body's natural detoxification processes and optimize their health and vitality from the inside out.

CHAPTER THREE

Dr. Barbara's Philosophy on Herbal Medicine and Detoxification

Dr. Barbara is a respected authority in the field of holistic health and wellness, renowned for her expertise in herbal medicine and detoxification. Central to her philosophy is the belief in the innate healing power of nature and the importance of supporting the body's natural detoxification processes to achieve optimal health and vitality. In this exploration, we delve into Dr. Barbara's philosophy on herbal medicine and detoxification, understanding her approach to holistic healing and wellness.

Holistic Approach to Health

At the core of Dr. Barbara's philosophy is a holistic approach to health that addresses the interconnectedness of the mind, body, and spirit. She believes that true health and wellness cannot be achieved by focusing solely on symptoms or isolated parts of the body but rather by considering the whole person and their unique constitution. Dr. Barbara recognizes that each individual is unique and may require personalized approaches to healing that take into account their physical, emotional, and spiritual well-being.

Healing Power of Nature

Dr. Barbara firmly believes in the healing power of nature and the abundant gifts it offers for promoting health and vitality. She draws inspiration from traditional healing systems such as Ayurveda, Traditional Chinese Medicine, and Native American herbalism, which have long recognized the therapeutic properties of plants and herbs. Dr. Barbara harnesses the wisdom of these ancient healing traditions and combines it with modern scientific research to create effective herbal formulations that support detoxification, balance the body, and promote overall well-being.

Supporting the Body's Natural Detoxification Processes

Detoxification is a cornerstone of Dr. Barbara's approach to health and wellness. She understands that in today's world, our bodies are constantly bombarded with toxins from environmental pollutants, processed foods, and stress, which can overwhelm the body's natural detoxification systems. Dr. Barbara's philosophy emphasizes the importance of supporting the liver, kidneys, digestive system, and other detox organs to effectively eliminate toxins and waste products from the body. She believes that by removing these obstacles to health, the body can restore balance and vitality, allowing individuals to experience optimal health and well-being.

Empowerment Through Education

Education is a key aspect of Dr. Barbara's philosophy, as she believes that empowered individuals are better equipped to take control of their health and make informed decisions about their well-being. Dr. Barbara provides comprehensive educational resources to her clients, including articles, videos, workshops, and personalized consultations, to help them understand the principles of herbal medicine, detoxification, and holistic health. By empowering individuals with knowledge and understanding, Dr. Barbara enables them to become active participants in their own healing journey.

Promoting Prevention and Long-Term Wellness

Dr. Barbara's philosophy extends beyond merely treating symptoms to focus on prevention and long-term wellness. She emphasizes the importance of lifestyle factors such as nutrition, exercise, stress management, and mindfulness practices in maintaining health and preventing disease. Dr. Barbara encourages her clients to adopt healthy habits that support their body's natural detoxification processes and promote overall well-being. By addressing the root causes of illness and imbalance, rather than merely masking symptoms, Dr. Barbara helps her clients achieve sustainable health and vitality for the long term.

Collaborative and Integrative Approach

Dr. Barbara takes a collaborative and integrative approach to health and wellness, working closely with her clients to develop personalized treatment plans that address their unique needs and goals. She recognizes the value of combining conventional and alternative therapies to achieve optimal results and often collaborates with other healthcare providers, including physicians, naturopaths, and holistic practitioners, to provide comprehensive care. Dr. Barbara understands that healing is a journey that requires support, guidance, and collaboration, and she is committed to empowering her clients every step of the way.

In conclusion, Dr. Barbara's philosophy on herbal medicine and detoxification is rooted in a holistic approach to health, the healing power of nature, supporting the body's natural detoxification processes, empowerment through education, promoting prevention and long-term wellness, and a collaborative and integrative approach to healing. By embracing these principles, Dr. Barbara helps her clients achieve optimal health and vitality, enabling them to live their best lives.

CHAPTER FOUR

The Power of Juicing: Extracting Nutrients for Cleansing

Juicing has long been hailed as a powerful tool for cleansing the body and extracting vital nutrients from fruits, vegetables, and herbs. In this exploration, we delve into the transformative potential of juicing, understanding how it facilitates detoxification and provides essential nutrients to support overall health and well-being.

Nutrient Extraction and Bioavailability

One of the primary benefits of juicing is its ability to extract concentrated nutrients from a variety of fresh produce. Fruits, vegetables, and herbs are rich sources of vitamins, minerals, antioxidants, and phytonutrients, which play essential roles in supporting the body's natural detoxification processes and promoting optimal health. Juicing allows for the rapid extraction of these nutrients in a form that is easily absorbed and utilized by the body, enhancing their bioavailability and maximizing their therapeutic benefits.

Promoting Detoxification

Juicing is an effective way to support the body's natural detoxification processes and promote cleansing from within. The concentrated nutrients found in fresh juices help nourish and support the liver, kidneys, digestive system, and other detox organs, enabling them to effectively eliminate toxins and waste products from the body. Juicing also provides hydration and alkalizing properties, which can help flush out toxins and restore balance to the body's internal environment. By supporting detoxification, juicing helps remove obstacles to health and vitality, allowing individuals to experience increased energy, clarity, and well-being.

Alkalizing and pH Balance

Many fruits and vegetables used in juicing are alkalizing to the body, meaning they help maintain a healthy pH balance and reduce acidity. An overly acidic environment in the body can contribute to inflammation, oxidative stress, and other health issues. Juicing alkalizing foods such as leafy greens, cucumber, celery, and lemon can help neutralize acidity, promote alkalinity, and support overall health and vitality. By consuming alkalizing juices regularly, individuals can create a more balanced internal environment, which is conducive to optimal health and well-being.

Hydration and Cellular Rejuvenation

Proper hydration is essential for overall health and well-being, and juicing provides a convenient and delicious way to stay hydrated while nourishing the body with essential nutrients. Fresh juices are rich in water, electrolytes, and hydration-promoting compounds, which help replenish fluids, support cellular hydration, and promote cellular rejuvenation. Hydrated cells are more efficient at detoxification and nutrient absorption, leading to increased energy, vitality, and overall well-being. Incorporating hydrating juices into one's daily routine is a simple yet powerful way to support cellular health and hydration from the inside out.

Antioxidant Support and Cellular Protection

Antioxidants are compounds found in fruits, vegetables, and herbs that help protect cells from damage caused by free radicals and oxidative stress. Juicing provides a concentrated source of antioxidants, including vitamins C and E, beta-carotene, and polyphenols, which help neutralize free radicals and promote cellular protection and repair. Antioxidant-rich juices help reduce inflammation, support immune function, and enhance the body's natural detoxification processes, leading to improved health and vitality. Regular consumption of antioxidant-rich juices can help individuals combat oxidative stress and promote longevity and well-being.

Supporting Digestive Health

Juicing can also support digestive health by providing a readily available source of enzymes, fiber, and prebiotics that promote optimal digestion and gut function. Enzymes help break down food and facilitate nutrient absorption, while fiber supports regularity and bowel health. Prebiotics nourish beneficial gut bacteria, promoting a healthy balance of microflora in the digestive tract. By supporting digestive health, juicing helps alleviate symptoms such as bloating, gas, and constipation, and promotes overall well-being. Incorporating fiber-rich vegetables such as kale, spinach, and carrots into juices can enhance their digestive benefits and support gut health.

In conclusion, juicing is a powerful tool for cleansing the body, extracting vital nutrients, and promoting overall health and well-being. By providing concentrated nutrients, promoting detoxification, alkalizing the body, supporting hydration, providing antioxidant protection, and supporting digestive health, juicing offers numerous benefits for health and vitality. Incorporating fresh juices into one's daily routine can help individuals achieve optimal health, energy, and vitality, allowing them to thrive and live their best lives.

CHAPTER FIVE

Essential Herbs for Detoxification and Refreshment

Detoxification is a natural process that the body undergoes to eliminate toxins and waste products, restoring balance and vitality. Herbs play a crucial role in supporting this process by providing a wide range of therapeutic benefits, including liver support, antioxidant protection, and digestive aid. In this exploration, we delve into some essential herbs for detoxification and refreshment, understanding their unique properties and how they can contribute to overall health and well-being.

1. Dandelion Root (Taraxacum officinale)

Dandelion root is a potent detoxifying herb that has been used for centuries in traditional medicine systems for its liver-cleansing properties. It contains compounds called sesquiterpene lactones, which stimulate bile production and flow, aiding in the elimination of toxins from the liver and gallbladder. Dandelion root also has diuretic properties, promoting the excretion of excess fluids and waste products from the body. Additionally, it is rich in antioxidants, vitamins, and minerals, which help protect cells from damage and support overall health and vitality.

2. Milk Thistle (Silybum marianum)

Milk thistle is renowned for its liver-protective and detoxifying properties, making it a valuable herb for supporting overall health and well-being. The active compound in milk thistle, silymarin, has powerful antioxidant and anti-inflammatory effects, which help protect the liver from damage caused by toxins and free radicals. Milk thistle also stimulates liver regeneration and enhances detoxification pathways, promoting the elimination of harmful substances from the body. By supporting liver health, milk thistle contributes to improved digestion, enhanced energy levels, and overall vitality.

3. Burdock Root (Arctium lappa)

Burdock root is a nourishing herb that supports detoxification and refreshment by promoting the elimination of toxins through the skin, kidneys, and lymphatic system. It contains a unique combination of prebiotic fibers, antioxidants, and anti-inflammatory compounds, which help cleanse the blood, support lymphatic drainage, and improve digestion. Burdock root also has diuretic properties, which aid in the elimination of excess fluids and waste products from the body. Additionally, it supports skin health and may help alleviate conditions such as acne, eczema, and psoriasis.

4. Ginger (Zingiber officinale)

Ginger is a warming herb with potent detoxifying and digestive properties, making it an excellent addition to detoxification protocols. It contains gingerol, a bioactive compound with antioxidant and anti-inflammatory effects, which help protect cells from damage and reduce inflammation in the body. Ginger also stimulates digestion, alleviates digestive discomfort, and promotes the elimination of toxins from the digestive tract. Its warming properties promote circulation and lymphatic drainage, supporting overall detoxification and rejuvenation.

5. Turmeric (Curcuma longa)

Turmeric is a powerhouse herb with numerous health benefits, including potent detoxifying and anti-inflammatory properties. It contains curcumin, a bioactive compound that has been extensively studied for its antioxidant, anti-inflammatory, and liver-protective effects. Turmeric helps support liver function, enhance bile production, and promote the elimination of toxins from the body. It also helps reduce inflammation, support immune function, and promote overall well-being. Incorporating turmeric into detoxification protocols can help support optimal health and vitality.

6. Nettle Leaf (Urtica dioica)

Nettle leaf is a nutrient-rich herb that supports detoxification and refreshment by promoting kidney function and urinary tract health. It has diuretic properties, which help increase urine production and promote the elimination of toxins and waste products from the body. Nettle leaf is also rich in vitamins, minerals, and antioxidants, which help nourish and support overall health and vitality. Additionally, it has anti-inflammatory effects, which help reduce inflammation in the body and promote optimal well-being.

7. Peppermint (Mentha piperita)

Peppermint is a refreshing herb with digestive and detoxifying properties, making it an excellent choice for supporting overall health and well-being. It contains menthol, a compound that helps relax the muscles of the digestive tract, alleviate digestive discomfort, and promote healthy digestion. Peppermint also has diuretic properties, which help promote the elimination of toxins through the urinary tract. Its refreshing aroma and flavor make it a popular choice for herbal teas and infused waters, providing a refreshing and invigorating experience.

In conclusion, these essential herbs for detoxification and refreshment play a crucial role in supporting the body's natural detoxification processes and promoting overall health and well-being. By incorporating these herbs into your diet and lifestyle, you can support optimal detoxification, enhance vitality, and experience a renewed sense of health and well-being.

CHAPTER SIX

Dr. Barbara's Herbal Juice Recipes for the 7-Day Detox

Dr. Barbara's Herbal Juice Recipes are specially formulated to support detoxification, nourish the body with essential nutrients, and promote overall well-being. These delicious and refreshing juices incorporate a variety of medicinal herbs and detoxifying ingredients to help cleanse the body, boost energy levels, and rejuvenate from within. Follow these recipes for a 7-day detox journey that will leave you feeling revitalized and refreshed.

Day 1: Green Cleanse Juice

Ingredients:

- 2 cups spinach
- 1 cucumber
- 2 stalks celery
- 1 green apple
- 1 inch ginger root
- 1 lemon (peeled)
- Handful of parsley

Instructions:

1. Wash all ingredients thoroughly.

2. Cut the cucumber, celery, and apple into smaller pieces for easier juicing.

3. Add all ingredients to a juicer and process until smooth.

4. Pour the juice into a glass and enjoy immediately.

Day 2: Liver Detox Elixir

Ingredients:

- 1 beetroot (peeled)

- 2 carrots

- 1 lemon (peeled)

- 1-inch turmeric root (or 1 tsp turmeric powder)

- 1-inch ginger root

- Handful of dandelion greens

Instructions:

1. Prepare all ingredients by washing and peeling if necessary.

2. Cut the beetroot, carrots, and lemon into smaller pieces.

3. Add all ingredients to a juicer and blend until smooth.

4. Pour the elixir into a glass and serve immediately.

Day 3: Cleansing Citrus Splash

Ingredients:

- 2 oranges (peeled)
- 1 grapefruit (peeled)
- 1 lemon (peeled)
- 1-inch ginger root
- Handful of mint leaves

Instructions:

1. Wash and peel the oranges, grapefruit, and lemon.

2. Cut the ginger into smaller pieces.

3. Juice all ingredients together in a juicer until well blended.

4. Garnish with fresh mint leaves and serve immediately.

Day 4: Refreshing Green Goddess

Ingredients:

- 2 cups kale
- 1 cucumber
- 1 green apple
- 1 pear
- 1 lemon (peeled)

- Handful of cilantro

Instructions:

1. Wash all ingredients thoroughly.

2. Cut the cucumber, apple, pear, and lemon into smaller pieces.

3. Juice all ingredients together in a juicer until smooth.

4. Pour into a glass and enjoy immediately.

Day 5: Antioxidant Berry Blast

Ingredients:

- 1 cup mixed berries (such as strawberries, blueberries, raspberries)

- 1 apple

- 1 cucumber

- Handful of spinach

- 1 lemon (peeled)

Instructions:

1. Wash all ingredients thoroughly.

2. Cut the apple and cucumber into smaller pieces.

3. Juice all ingredients together in a blender until well blended.

4. Pour into a glass and serve immediately.

Day 6: Immune-Boosting Turmeric Tonic

Ingredients:

- 1 orange (peeled)
- 1 lemon (peeled)
- 1-inch turmeric root (or 1 tsp turmeric powder)
- 1-inch ginger root
- Pinch of black pepper (to enhance turmeric absorption)

Instructions:

1. Wash and peel the orange and lemon.
2. Cut the turmeric and ginger into smaller pieces.
3. Juice all ingredients together in a juicer until smooth.
4. Add a pinch of black pepper and stir well before serving.

Day 7: Detoxifying Herbal Infusion

Ingredients:

- 1 liter water
- 1 cucumber (sliced)
- 1 lemon (sliced)

- Handful of fresh mint leaves

- Handful of fresh basil leaves

- 1-inch ginger root (sliced)

- Optional: a few slices of fresh turmeric root

Instructions:

1. Bring the water to a boil in a large pot.

2. Add all the ingredients to the boiling water.

3. Reduce the heat and let the infusion simmer for 10-15 minutes.

4. Remove from heat and let it cool slightly.

5. Strain the mixture and transfer the infused water to a pitcher.

6. Refrigerate until chilled.

7. Serve the herbal infusion over ice and garnish with additional mint leaves if desired.

These herbal juice recipes are designed to support detoxification, nourish the body with essential nutrients, and promote overall well-being. Incorporate them into your 7-day detox journey for a refreshing and rejuvenating experience that will leave you feeling revitalized from the inside out.

CHAPTER SEVEN

Incorporating Alkaline Foods for Enhanced Detoxification

Alkaline foods play a crucial role in supporting enhanced detoxification by promoting a more alkaline environment in the body. These foods are rich in alkalizing minerals such as potassium, magnesium, and calcium, which help neutralize acidity and reduce inflammation. By incorporating alkaline foods into your diet, you can support the body's natural detoxification processes and promote overall health and well-being. Here's how to incorporate alkaline foods for enhanced detoxification:

1. Leafy Greens

Leafy greens such as kale, spinach, Swiss chard, and collard greens are excellent alkaline foods that are rich in chlorophyll, vitamins, minerals, and antioxidants. These nutrient-dense greens help alkalize the body and support detoxification by promoting liver function, enhancing digestion, and reducing inflammation. Incorporate leafy greens into your daily diet by adding them to salads, smoothies, juices, soups, and stir-fries.

2. Cruciferous Vegetables

Cruciferous vegetables like broccoli, cauliflower, Brussels sprouts, and cabbage are alkaline foods that are high in fiber, vitamins, minerals, and phytonutrients. These vegetables contain compounds called glucosinolates, which support liver detoxification and promote the elimination of toxins from the body. Include cruciferous vegetables in your meals by steaming, roasting, or sautéing them as a side dish or adding them to soups, salads, and stir-fries.

3. Citrus Fruits

Citrus fruits such as lemons, limes, oranges, and grapefruits are alkaline-forming foods that are rich in vitamin C, antioxidants, and electrolytes. Despite their acidic taste, citrus fruits have an alkalizing effect on the body once metabolized. They help support liver function, aid digestion, and promote hydration, making them ideal for enhancing detoxification. Start your day with a glass of warm lemon water or incorporate citrus fruits into salads, smoothies, juices, and desserts.

4. Root Vegetables

Root vegetables like carrots, beets, sweet potatoes, and radishes are alkaline foods that are rich in fiber, vitamins, minerals, and antioxidants. These vegetables help alkalize the body and support detoxification by promoting liver function, improving digestion, and boosting immune function. Incorporate root vegetables into your meals by roasting, steaming, or baking them as a side dish or adding them to soups, stews, salads, and Buddha bowls.

5. Herbs and Spices

Herbs and spices such as ginger, turmeric, cinnamon, and cilantro are alkaline-forming foods that are rich in antioxidants, anti-inflammatory compounds, and essential nutrients. These flavorful additions help alkalize the body and support detoxification by promoting liver function, aiding digestion, and reducing inflammation. Incorporate herbs and spices into your meals by adding them to soups, stews, stir-fries, salads, smoothies, and herbal teas.

6. Nuts and Seeds

Nuts and seeds such as almonds, walnuts, chia seeds, and flaxseeds are alkaline-forming foods that are rich in healthy fats, protein, fiber, vitamins, minerals, and antioxidants. These nutrient-dense foods help alkalize the body and support detoxification by promoting liver function, reducing inflammation, and supporting cellular health. Incorporate nuts and seeds into your diet by adding them to salads, smoothies, oatmeal, yogurt, and homemade energy bars.

7. Alkaline Water and Herbal Teas

In addition to alkaline foods, incorporating alkaline water and herbal teas into your daily routine can further support detoxification and promote hydration. Alkaline water has a higher pH level than regular water, which helps neutralize acidity in the body and support optimal hydration. Herbal teas such as dandelion root tea, ginger tea, and peppermint tea have alkalizing properties and can help support liver function, aid digestion, and promote overall well-being.

By incorporating alkaline foods into your diet, you can support enhanced detoxification, promote alkalinity in the body, and experience improved health and vitality. Start by incorporating a variety of leafy greens, cruciferous vegetables, citrus fruits, root vegetables, herbs, spices, nuts, seeds, alkaline water, and herbal teas into your meals and snacks to support your body's natural detoxification processes and promote overall well-being.

CHAPTER EIGHT

Hydration and Supplements for Optimal Detox Results

Hydration and supplementation play crucial roles in supporting optimal detoxification results by facilitating the elimination of toxins, replenishing essential nutrients, and promoting overall health and well-being. In this guide, we'll explore the importance of hydration and supplementation in detox programs and discuss strategies for incorporating them into your routine for maximum effectiveness.

Hydration: The Foundation of Detoxification

Proper hydration is essential for supporting the body's natural detoxification processes. Water plays a vital role in flushing out toxins, transporting nutrients, and maintaining cellular function. During detoxification, the body needs even more water to support the increased elimination of toxins through urine, sweat, and bowel movements.

Tips for Staying Hydrated During Detox:

1. **Drink Plenty of Water:** Aim to drink at least 8-10 glasses of water per day, or more if you're engaging in vigorous exercise or sweating heavily.

2. **Incorporate Herbal Teas:** Herbal teas such as dandelion root tea, ginger tea, and green tea can support hydration while providing additional detoxifying benefits.

3. **Add Electrolytes:** Consider adding electrolyte-rich foods and beverages such as coconut water, cucumber, and watermelon to your diet to help replenish electrolytes lost during detox.

4. **Avoid Dehydrating Beverages:** Minimize or avoid beverages such as alcohol, caffeinated drinks, and sugary sodas, which can dehydrate the body and hinder detoxification efforts.

5. **Monitor Urine Color:** Aim for pale yellow urine, which indicates adequate hydration. Darker urine may indicate dehydration and a need to increase fluid intake.

Supplements to Support Detoxification:

In addition to hydration, certain supplements can enhance the detoxification process by providing targeted support to the liver, kidneys, and other detox organs. These supplements help optimize detoxification pathways, neutralize free radicals, and promote overall health and well-being.

Key Supplements for Detoxification:

1. **Milk Thistle:** Milk thistle is a potent liver-supportive herb that contains the active compound silymarin, which helps protect liver cells from damage and promotes detoxification.

2. **N-Acetyl Cysteine (NAC):** NAC is a precursor to glutathione, a powerful antioxidant and detoxifier produced by the liver. Supplementing with NAC can support glutathione production and enhance detoxification.

3. **Alpha-Lipoic Acid (ALA):** ALA is a powerful antioxidant that helps regenerate other antioxidants such as glutathione and vitamin C. It also supports liver function and detoxification.

4. **Chlorella and Spirulina:** These nutrient-dense algae are rich in chlorophyll, vitamins, minerals, and antioxidants, which help support detoxification, promote cellular health, and boost energy levels.

5. **Probiotics:** Probiotics help support gut health and promote the growth of beneficial bacteria in the digestive tract. A healthy gut microbiome is essential for proper digestion, nutrient absorption, and detoxification.

6. **Magnesium:** Magnesium plays a crucial role in over 300 biochemical reactions in the body, including detoxification processes. Supplementing with magnesium can support muscle relaxation, stress reduction, and detoxification.

Tips for Supplement Use During Detox:

1. **Consult with a Healthcare Professional:** Before starting any new supplement regimen, consult with a qualified

healthcare professional to ensure it's appropriate for your individual needs and health status.

2. **Choose High-Quality Supplements:** Look for supplements that are third-party tested for quality, purity, and potency to ensure you're getting the most effective and bioavailable forms of nutrients.

3. **Follow Recommended Dosages:** Stick to the recommended dosages provided by the manufacturer or your healthcare provider to avoid potential side effects or interactions with other medications.

4. **Monitor Your Body's Response:** Pay attention to how your body responds to supplements and make adjustments as needed. If you experience any adverse reactions, discontinue use and consult with your healthcare provider.

In conclusion, hydration and supplementation are essential components of any detox program, supporting the body's natural detoxification processes and promoting overall health and well-being. By staying hydrated, incorporating targeted supplements, and consulting with a healthcare professional, you can optimize your detoxification efforts and achieve optimal results.

CHAPTER NINE

Addressing Detox Symptoms and Challenges

Embarking on a detoxification journey can bring about various symptoms and challenges as the body undergoes the process of eliminating toxins and adjusting to dietary and lifestyle changes. Understanding and effectively managing these symptoms is essential for a successful and comfortable detox experience. In this guide, we'll explore common detox symptoms and challenges and provide strategies for addressing them.

1. Common Detox Symptoms:

- **Fatigue and Lethargy:** As the body works to eliminate toxins, it may experience temporary fatigue and lethargy. This can be exacerbated by changes in diet, reduced calorie intake, and increased physical activity.

- **Headaches:** Headaches are a common detox symptom and can be caused by dehydration, caffeine withdrawal, or the release of toxins from fat cells. They usually subside as the detox progresses.

- **Digestive Issues:** Detoxification can temporarily disrupt digestive function, leading to symptoms such as bloating, gas, constipation, or diarrhea. This can occur as the body adjusts to dietary changes and eliminates toxins.

- **Skin Breakouts:** The skin is a major detoxification organ, and as toxins are eliminated from the body, they can sometimes manifest as skin breakouts or rashes. This is often temporary and resolves as the detox progresses.

2. Strategies for Addressing Detox Symptoms:

- **Stay Hydrated:** Proper hydration is essential for supporting the body's detoxification processes and minimizing symptoms such as fatigue, headaches, and digestive issues. Drink plenty of water throughout the day and incorporate hydrating herbal teas and electrolyte-rich beverages.

- **Gradual Transition:** Ease into your detox program gradually to minimize detox symptoms and allow your body to adjust more comfortably. Start by eliminating processed foods, caffeine, alcohol, and sugar, and gradually increase your intake of whole foods, fruits, vegetables, and herbal teas.

- **Support Liver Health:** The liver plays a central role in detoxification, so supporting liver function can help alleviate detox symptoms. Incorporate liver-supportive herbs such as milk thistle, dandelion root, and turmeric into your detox regimen to promote liver detoxification and support overall health.

- **Manage Stress:** Stress can exacerbate detox symptoms and hinder the body's ability to detoxify effectively. Practice stress-reducing techniques such as deep breathing, meditation, yoga, or gentle exercise to promote relaxation and support overall well-being during the detox process.

- **Include Nutrient-Dense Foods:** Ensure that your detox diet includes a variety of nutrient-dense foods to provide essential vitamins, minerals, antioxidants, and phytonutrients that support detoxification and overall health. Include plenty of leafy greens, cruciferous vegetables, fruits, nuts, seeds, and lean proteins in your meals.

- **Listen to Your Body:** Pay attention to your body's signals and adjust your detox program as needed. If you experience severe or persistent symptoms, consider modifying your detox protocol, consulting with a healthcare professional, or discontinuing the detox altogether if necessary.

3. Long-Term Detox Challenges:

- **Cravings and Temptations:** Managing cravings for unhealthy foods and resisting temptation can be challenging during and after a detox program. Stay focused on your goals, practice mindful eating, and have healthy snacks on hand to satisfy cravings.

- **Sustainability:** Maintaining the benefits of a detox program in the long term can be challenging. Focus on incorporating healthy habits into your daily routine, such as eating a balanced diet, staying hydrated, exercising regularly, managing stress, and getting enough sleep.

- **Social Pressures:** Social situations and peer pressure can sometimes make it difficult to stick to a detox program or healthy lifestyle changes. Communicate your goals with friends and family, seek support from like-minded individuals, and make conscious choices that align with your health priorities.

- **Emotional Challenges:** Detoxification can sometimes bring up emotional challenges as well, such as mood swings, irritability, or emotional detoxification. Practice self-care, engage in activities that bring you joy and relaxation, and seek support from friends, family, or a professional if needed.

In conclusion, addressing detox symptoms and challenges requires a combination of strategies, including staying hydrated, supporting liver health, managing stress, incorporating nutrient-dense foods, listening to your body, and addressing long-term challenges such as cravings, sustainability, social pressures, and emotional well-being. By taking a holistic approach to detoxification and focusing on supporting your body's natural detoxification processes, you can achieve optimal results and maintain long-term health and vitality.

CHAPTER TEN

Long-Term Health Maintenance: Post-Detox Guidelines and Lifestyle Changes

Completing a detox program is just the first step towards achieving long-term health and vitality. To maintain the benefits of your detox and continue on a path of wellness, it's important to implement post-detox guidelines and make sustainable lifestyle changes. In this guide, we'll outline post-detox guidelines and lifestyle changes to support your ongoing health maintenance.

1. Gradual Transition:

After completing a detox program, it's essential to transition back to a regular diet gradually. Reintroduce foods slowly, starting with easily digestible foods such as fruits, vegetables, and whole grains. Avoid processed foods, refined sugars, caffeine, and alcohol, as these can undo the benefits of your detox and lead to energy crashes and cravings.

2. Balanced Nutrition:

Focus on maintaining a balanced and nutrient-dense diet rich in fruits, vegetables, whole grains, lean proteins, and healthy fats. Aim to include a variety of colors and textures in your meals to ensure you're getting a wide range of vitamins, minerals, antioxidants, and phytonutrients. Incorporate foods that support detoxification, such as leafy greens, cruciferous vegetables, herbs, spices, and antioxidant-rich fruits.

3. Hydration:

Continue to prioritize hydration by drinking plenty of water throughout the day. Aim for at least 8-10 glasses of water daily, or more if you're physically active or live in a hot climate. Hydration supports detoxification, aids digestion, promotes cellular health, and helps maintain energy levels and overall well-being. Consider incorporating hydrating beverages such as herbal teas, coconut water, and infused water with fresh fruits and herbs.

4. Regular Exercise:

Engage in regular physical activity to support overall health and vitality. Exercise helps stimulate circulation, promote detoxification, reduce stress, support weight management, and boost mood and energy levels. Find activities you enjoy, whether it's walking, jogging, cycling, yoga, dancing, swimming, or strength training, and aim for at least 30 minutes of moderate-intensity exercise most days of the week.

5. Stress Management:

Prioritize stress management techniques to support your overall well-being. Chronic stress can negatively impact detoxification, digestion, immune function, and mental health. Practice stress-reducing activities such as deep breathing, meditation, mindfulness, yoga, tai chi, or spending time in nature. Establish healthy boundaries, prioritize self-care, and seek support from friends, family, or a professional if needed.

6. Quality Sleep:

Ensure you're getting adequate and restorative sleep each night to support detoxification, hormone balance, immune function, and overall health. Aim for 7-9 hours of quality sleep in a dark, quiet, and comfortable environment. Establish a consistent sleep schedule, practice relaxing bedtime rituals, limit screen time before bed, and create a sleep-friendly bedroom environment to optimize sleep quality.

7. Mindful Eating:

Practice mindful eating to cultivate a healthy relationship with food and support digestion, nutrient absorption, and overall well-being. Pay attention to hunger and fullness cues, eat slowly, savor each bite, and chew your food thoroughly. Choose whole, minimally processed foods, and eat with intention, focusing on nourishing your body and honoring its needs.

8. Regular Detox Maintenance:

Incorporate regular detox maintenance practices into your lifestyle to support ongoing detoxification and overall health. This may include periodic cleanses, fasting, juice fasts, herbal teas, sauna sessions, dry brushing, lymphatic massage, or other detox-supportive practices. Consult with a healthcare professional before starting any new detox program or practice.

By implementing these post-detox guidelines and lifestyle changes, you can maintain the benefits of your detox program, support your ongoing health and vitality, and cultivate a sustainable approach to wellness for the long term. Remember that consistency and balance are key, and small, gradual changes over time can lead to significant improvements in your health and well-being.

CHAPTER 11

DR. BARBARA JUICE RECIPES FOR FULL-BODY DETOX

1. Green Goddess Detox Juice

- **Definition:** This juice is packed with green veggies and fruits known for their detoxifying properties.

- **Ingredients:** Spinach, kale, cucumber, green apple, celery, lemon, ginger.

- **How to Prepare:** Wash all the ingredients thoroughly. Chop them into smaller pieces. Run them through a juicer.

- **How to Use:** Drink a glass of this juice in the morning on an empty stomach.

- **Dosage:** One glass daily.

- **Side Effects:** Unlikely, but individuals with kidney issues should consult a doctor due to the high oxalate content in spinach and kale.

- **Precautions:** Monitor blood sugar levels if diabetic due to the natural sugars in the fruits.

2. Citrus Carrot Cleanse Juice

- **Definition:** A refreshing juice blend rich in vitamin C and beta-carotene for detoxifying and rejuvenating.

- **Ingredients:** Oranges, carrots, lemon, turmeric.

- **How to Prepare:** Peel the oranges, wash the carrots and lemon. Cut into smaller pieces. Juice them together with turmeric.

- **How to Use:** Best consumed in the morning or as a midday pick-me-up.

- **Dosage:** One glass daily.

- **Side Effects:** None reported, but excessive intake of turmeric may cause digestive discomfort in some.

- **Precautions:** Avoid if allergic to any of the ingredients.

3. Beetroot Cleanse Juice

- **Definition:** Beetroot is known for its detoxifying properties and helps in cleansing the liver.

- **Ingredients:** Beetroot, apple, carrot, ginger, lemon.

- **How to Prepare:** Wash and peel the beetroot, apple, carrot, and ginger. Cut into smaller pieces. Juice them together with lemon.

- **How to Use:** Consume this juice in the morning before breakfast.

- **Dosage:** One glass daily.

- **Side Effects:** Beetroot may cause red or pink urine, which is harmless.

- **Precautions:** Excessive consumption may lead to beeturia (passing red or pink urine).

4. **Pineapple Mint Detox Juice**

- **Definition:** A tropical juice blend with pineapple and mint for a refreshing detoxifying experience.

- **Ingredients:** Pineapple, cucumber, mint leaves, lime.

- **How to Prepare:** Peel the pineapple, wash the cucumber and mint. Cut into smaller pieces. Juice them together with lime.

- **How to Use:** Enjoy this juice as a midday refresher.

- **Dosage:** One glass daily.

- **Side Effects:** Unlikely, but excessive consumption of pineapple may cause mouth or throat irritation.

- **Precautions:** Avoid if allergic to any of the ingredients.

5. **Watermelon Detox Juice**

- **Definition:** Watermelon is hydrating and contains antioxidants that aid in detoxification.

- **Ingredients:** Watermelon, cucumber, lime, basil.

- **How to Prepare:** Remove seeds from watermelon, wash cucumber and basil, and cut into smaller pieces. Juice them together with lime.

- **How to Use:** Best enjoyed as a refreshing drink on a hot day.

- **Dosage:** One glass daily.

- **Side Effects:** None reported, but excessive consumption may cause digestive upset due to its high water content.

- **Precautions:** Monitor blood sugar levels if diabetic due to natural sugars in watermelon.

6. Turmeric Spice Detox Juice

- **Definition:** Turmeric is known for its anti-inflammatory and detoxifying properties.

- **Ingredients:** Carrot, apple, turmeric root, lemon, black pepper.

- **How to Prepare:** Wash carrot, apple, and lemon. Peel turmeric root. Cut into smaller pieces. Juice them together with black pepper.

- **How to Use:** Consume this juice in the morning or as a pre-workout drink.

- **Dosage:** One glass daily.

- **Side Effects:** Excessive intake of turmeric may cause gastrointestinal issues in some individuals.

- **Precautions:** Avoid if allergic to any of the ingredients.

7. Cranberry Detox Juice

- **Definition:** Cranberries are known for their detoxifying and urinary tract health benefits.

- **Ingredients:** Cranberries, cucumber, apple, lemon, ginger.

- **How to Prepare:** Wash all ingredients. Cut into smaller pieces. Juice them together.

- **How to Use:** Best consumed in the morning on an empty stomach.

- **Dosage:** One glass daily.

- **Side Effects:** Excessive consumption may cause gastrointestinal upset or diarrhea.

- **Precautions:** Avoid if prone to kidney stones due to the high oxalate content in cranberries.

8. Ginger Lemon Cleanse Juice

- **Definition:** A simple yet powerful detox juice that aids digestion and supports liver health.

- **Ingredients:** Ginger, lemon, apple, cucumber, spinach.

- **How to Prepare:** Wash all ingredients. Peel ginger and lemon if desired. Cut into smaller pieces. Juice them together.

- **How to Use:** Consume this juice in the morning before breakfast.

- **Dosage:** One glass daily.

- **Side Effects:** Excessive ginger consumption may cause heartburn or digestive discomfort in some individuals.

- **Precautions:** Monitor blood sugar levels if diabetic due to natural sugars in fruits.

9. Kale Pineapple Detox Juice

- **Definition:** Kale is a nutrient-dense green that aids in detoxification and pineapple adds a tropical twist.

- **Ingredients:** Kale, pineapple, cucumber, lemon, ginger.

- **How to Prepare:** Wash kale, pineapple, cucumber, and lemon. Cut into smaller pieces. Juice them together with ginger.

- **How to Use:** Enjoy this juice in the morning or as a post-workout drink.

- **Dosage:** One glass daily.

- **Side Effects:** None reported, but excessive kale consumption may interfere with blood clotting in some individuals.

- **Precautions:** Avoid if allergic to any of the ingredients.

10. Aloe Vera Detox Juice

- **Definition:** Aloe vera is known for its detoxifying and gut-soothing properties.

- **Ingredients:** Aloe vera gel, cucumber, apple, lemon, mint.

- **How to Prepare:** Extract gel from aloe vera leaf. Wash cucumber, apple, lemon, and mint. Cut into smaller pieces. Juice them together with aloe vera gel.

- **How to Use:** Consume this juice in the morning on an empty stomach.

- **Dosage:** One glass daily.

- **Side Effects:** Excessive intake of aloe vera may cause diarrhea or gastrointestinal discomfort.

- **Precautions:** Use only the gel portion of aloe vera leaf, as the outer skin can be toxic if ingested.

11.   Mango Papaya Cleanse Juice

- **Definition:** Mango and papaya are tropical fruits rich in enzymes that aid digestion and detoxification.

- **Ingredients:** Mango, papaya, pineapple, lime, mint.

- **How to Prepare:** Peel mango and papaya, wash pineapple, lime, and mint. Cut into smaller pieces. Juice them together.

- **How to Use:** Best enjoyed as a refreshing drink in the morning.

- **Dosage:** One glass daily.

- **Side Effects:** None reported, but excessive consumption may cause gastrointestinal upset due to high fiber content.

- **Precautions:** Avoid if allergic to any of the ingredients.

12.   Celery Cucumber Cleanse Juice

- **Definition:** Celery and cucumber are hydrating vegetables with natural diuretic properties that aid in detoxification.

- **Ingredients:** Celery, cucumber, lemon, parsley.

- **How to Prepare:** Wash all ingredients. Cut into smaller pieces. Juice them together.

- **How to Use:** Consume this juice in the morning or as a pre-meal appetizer.

- **Dosage:** One glass daily.

- **Side Effects:** Excessive intake may cause electrolyte imbalance due to the diuretic properties.

- **Precautions:** Monitor electrolyte levels if consuming large quantities.

13. **Spinach Berry Detox Juice**

- **Definition:** Spinach is rich in antioxidants and berries add a burst of flavor and additional nutrients.

- **Ingredients:** Spinach, mixed berries (strawberries, blueberries, raspberries), cucumber, lemon, ginger.

- **How to Prepare:** Wash spinach, berries, and cucumber. Cut into smaller pieces. Juice them together with lemon and ginger.

- **How to Use:** Best consumed in the morning or as a post-workout drink.

- **Dosage:** One glass daily.

- **Side Effects:** Unlikely, but excessive spinach consumption may interfere with blood clotting in some individuals.

- **Precautions:** Avoid if allergic to any of the ingredients.

14. **Carrot Ginger Cleanse Juice**

- **Definition:** Carrots are rich in beta-carotene and ginger aids digestion and reduces inflammation.

- **Ingredients:** Carrot, ginger, apple, lemon, turmeric.

- **How to Prepare:** Wash all ingredients. Peel carrot, ginger, and lemon if desired. Cut into smaller pieces. Juice them together with turmeric.

- **How to Use:** Consume this juice in the morning or as a pre-meal appetizer.

- **Dosage:** One glass daily.

- **Side Effects:** Excessive ginger intake may cause heartburn or digestive discomfort.

- **Precautions:** Monitor blood sugar levels if diabetic due to natural sugars in fruits.

15.   Pomegranate Beet Cleanse Juice

- **Definition:** Pomegranate and beetroot combine to create a vibrant detox juice rich in antioxidants and vitamins.

- **Ingredients:** Pomegranate seeds, beetroot, cucumber, lemon, ginger.

- **How to Prepare:** Deseed pomegranate, wash beetroot, cucumber, and lemon. Cut into smaller pieces. Juice them together with ginger.

- **How to Use:** Enjoy this juice as a midday refresher or post-workout drink.

- **Dosage:** One glass daily.

- **Side Effects:** Beetroot may cause red or pink urine, which is harmless.

- **Precautions:** Excessive consumption may lead to beeturia (passing red or pink urine).

SOME VITAL HERBAL REMEDIES TO KNOW

Agrimony:

Definition: Agrimony, scientifically known as Agrimonia eupatoria, is a perennial herbaceous plant native to Europe, Asia, and North America. It has a long history of use in traditional medicine, particularly in European folk medicine, for its potential health benefits.

Ingredients: Agrimony contains various bioactive compounds, including tannins, flavonoids, phenolic acids, and volatile oils. These compounds are believed to contribute to the herb's medicinal properties, including its potential as an astringent, anti-inflammatory, and digestive aid.

How to Prepare: Agrimony is typically prepared and consumed as an herbal tea, tincture, or poultice. To make tea, dried agrimony leaves and flowers are steeped in hot water for several minutes before being strained and consumed. Tinctures are prepared by steeping the herb in alcohol or vinegar to extract its active compounds.

Dosage: The appropriate dosage of agrimony can vary depending on factors such as age, health status, and the specific preparation being used. It's important to follow the recommended dosage on the product label or consult with a qualified herbalist or healthcare professional for personalized guidance.

How to Use: Agrimony tea, tincture, or poultice is typically taken orally or applied topically. It's often consumed to soothe gastrointestinal issues, such as indigestion and diarrhea, or used externally to treat skin conditions.

Side Effects: Agrimony is generally considered safe for most people when used in moderate amounts. However, some individuals may experience allergic reactions or gastrointestinal upset. It may also interact with certain medications or have adverse effects in individuals with certain health conditions. It's important to use agrimony under the guidance of a healthcare professional and to discontinue use if any adverse effects occur.

Alfalfa:

Definition: Alfalfa, scientifically known as Medicago sativa, is a flowering plant in the pea family native to Asia but cultivated worldwide. It's primarily grown as fodder for livestock, but it has also been used in traditional medicine for its potential health benefits.

Ingredients: Alfalfa contains various bioactive compounds, including vitamins (such as vitamin A, vitamin C, and vitamin K), minerals (including calcium, magnesium, and potassium), amino acids, and phytoestrogens. These compounds are believed to contribute to the herb's medicinal properties, including its potential as a nutritive tonic, diuretic, and hormone balancer.

How to Prepare: Alfalfa is typically consumed as sprouts, herbal tea, or in supplement form (such as capsules or tablets). To make tea, dried alfalfa leaves are steeped in hot water for several minutes before being strained and consumed.

Dosage: The appropriate dosage of alfalfa can vary depending on factors such as age, health status, and the specific preparation being used. It's important to follow the recommended dosage on the product label or consult with a qualified herbalist or healthcare professional for personalized guidance.

How to Use: Alfalfa sprouts, tea, or supplements are typically taken orally. It's often consumed as a dietary supplement to support overall health and well-being, as well as to promote kidney health and hormone balance.

Side Effects: Alfalfa is generally considered safe for most people when consumed in moderate amounts. However, some individuals may experience allergic reactions or digestive upset. It may also interact with certain medications or have adverse effects in individuals with certain health conditions, such as autoimmune diseases or hormone-sensitive conditions. Pregnant or breastfeeding individuals should consult with a healthcare professional before using alfalfa supplements. It's important to use alfalfa under the guidance of a healthcare professional and to discontinue use if any adverse effects occur.

Ashwagandha:

Definition: Ashwagandha, scientifically known as Withaniasomnifera, is a small shrub native to India, the Middle East, and parts of Africa. It has a long history of use in Ayurvedic medicine for its potential health benefits, particularly for its adaptogenic properties.

Ingredients: Ashwagandha root contains various bioactive compounds, including alkaloids (such as withanolides), steroidal lactones, and flavonoids. These compounds are believed to contribute to the herb's medicinal properties, including its potential as an adaptogen, anti-inflammatory, and immune-modulating agent.

How to Prepare: Ashwagandha is typically consumed as a powdered root, herbal tea, tincture, or in supplement form (such as capsules or tablets). To make tea, dried ashwagandha root is steeped in hot water for several minutes before being strained and consumed.

Dosage: The appropriate dosage of ashwagandha can vary depending on factors such as age, health status, and the specific preparation being used. It's important to follow the recommended dosage on the product label or consult with a qualified herbalist or healthcare professional for personalized guidance.

How to Use: Ashwagandha powder, tea, tincture, or supplements are typically taken orally. It's often consumed to support stress management, promote relaxation, and boost overall vitality and well-being.

Side Effects: Ashwagandha is generally considered safe for most people when used in moderate amounts. However, some individuals may experience mild side effects such as gastrointestinal upset or drowsiness. It may also interact with certain medications or have adverse effects in individuals with certain health conditions, such as autoimmune diseases or thyroid disorders. Pregnant or breastfeeding individuals should consult with a healthcare professional before using ashwagandha supplements. It's important to use ashwagandha under the guidance of a healthcare professional and to discontinue use if any adverse effects occur.

Astragalus:

Definition: Astragalus, scientifically known as Astragalus membranaceus, is a flowering plant native to China and Mongolia but also found in other parts of Asia. It has been used for centuries in traditional Chinese medicine for its potential health benefits, particularly for its immune-enhancing properties.

Ingredients: Astragalus root contains various bioactive compounds, including polysaccharides, saponins (such as astragalosides), flavonoids, and amino acids. These compounds are believed to contribute to the herb's medicinal properties, including its potential as an adaptogen, immunomodulator, and anti-inflammatory agent.

How to Prepare: Astragalus is typically consumed as a powdered root, herbal tea, tincture, or in supplement form (such as capsules or tablets). To make tea, dried astragalus root slices are simmered in water for several minutes before being strained and consumed.

Dosage: The appropriate dosage of astragalus can vary depending on factors such as age, health status, and the specific preparation being used. It's important to follow the recommended dosage on the product label or consult with a qualified herbalist or healthcare professional for personalized guidance.

How to Use: Astragalus powder, tea, tincture, or supplements are typically taken orally. It's often consumed to support immune function, promote vitality, and enhance overall well-being.

Side Effects: Astragalus is generally considered safe for most people when used in moderate amounts. However, some individuals may experience mild side effects such as gastrointestinal upset or allergic reactions. It may also interact with certain medications or have adverse effects in individuals with certain health conditions, such as autoimmune diseases or diabetes. Pregnant or breastfeeding individuals should consult with a healthcare professional before using astragalus supplements. It's important to use astragalus under the guidance of a healthcare professional and to discontinue use if any adverse effects occur.

Black Cohosh:

Definition: Black cohosh, scientifically known as Actaea racemosa (formerly Cimicifuga racemosa), is a perennial herb native to North America. It has a long history of use in traditional Native American medicine and later in folk medicine for its potential health benefits, particularly for women's health.

Ingredients: Black cohosh root contains various bioactive compounds, including triterpene glycosides (such as actein and cimicifugoside), phenolic acids, and flavonoids. These compounds are believed to contribute to the herb's medicinal properties, including its potential as a hormone-balancing agent and its ability to relieve menopausal symptoms.

How to Prepare: Black cohosh is typically consumed as a powdered root, herbal tea, tincture, or in supplement form (such as capsules or tablets). To make tea, dried black cohosh root is steeped in hot water for several minutes before being strained and consumed.

Dosage: The appropriate dosage of black cohosh can vary depending on factors such as age, health status, and the specific preparation being used. It's important to follow the recommended dosage on the product label or consult with a qualified herbalist or healthcare professional for personalized guidance.

How to Use: Black cohosh powder, tea, tincture, or supplements are typically taken orally. It's often used by women to support hormonal balance, relieve menopausal symptoms such as hot flashes and night sweats, and promote overall well-being.

Side Effects: Black cohosh is generally considered safe for most people when used in moderate amounts. However, some individuals may experience mild side effects such as gastrointestinal upset or allergic reactions. It may also interact with certain medications or have adverse effects in individuals with certain health conditions, such as liver disease or hormone-sensitive conditions. Pregnant or breastfeeding individuals should consult with a healthcare professional before using black cohosh supplements. It's important to use black cohosh under the guidance of a healthcare professional and to discontinue use if any adverse effects occur.

Cat's Claw:

Definition: Cat's claw, scientifically known as Uncaria tomentosa, is a woody vine native to the Amazon rainforest and other parts of Central and South America. It has been used for centuries in traditional medicine by indigenous peoples for its potential health benefits.

Ingredients: Cat's claw contains various bioactive compounds, including alkaloids (such as oxindole alkaloids and quinovic acid glycosides), polyphenols, and other phytochemicals. These compounds are believed to contribute to the herb's medicinal properties, including its potential as an immune enhancer, anti-inflammatory, and antioxidant.

How to Prepare: Cat's claw is typically consumed as an herbal tea, tincture, or in supplement form (such as capsules or tablets). To make tea, dried cat's claw bark or leaves are steeped in hot water for several minutes before being strained and consumed.

Dosage: The appropriate dosage of cat's claw can vary depending on factors such as age, health status, and the specific preparation being used. It's important to follow the recommended dosage on the product label or consult with a qualified herbalist or healthcare professional for personalized guidance.

How to Use: Cat's claw tea, tincture, or supplements are typically taken orally. It's often used to support immune function, reduce inflammation, and promote overall well-being.

Side Effects: Cat's claw is generally considered safe for most people when used in moderate amounts. However, some individuals may experience mild side effects such as gastrointestinal upset or allergic reactions. It may also interact with certain medications or have adverse effects in individuals with certain health conditions, such as autoimmune diseases or bleeding disorders. Pregnant or breastfeeding individuals should consult with a healthcare professional before using cat's claw supplements. It's important to use cat's claw under the guidance of a healthcare professional and to discontinue use if any adverse effects occur.

Chickweed:

Definition: Chickweed, scientifically known as Stellaria media, is an annual herbaceous plant native to Europe but naturalized in many other parts of the world. It's often considered a common weed but has been used historically in traditional medicine for its potential health benefits.

Ingredients: Chickweed contains various bioactive compounds, including flavonoids, saponins, mucilage, and vitamins (such as vitamin C). These compounds are believed to contribute to the herb's medicinal properties, including its potential as a demulcent, anti-inflammatory, and mild diuretic.

How to Prepare: Chickweed is typically consumed as an herbal tea, infusion, or in fresh salads. To make tea, dried chickweed leaves and flowers are steeped in hot water for several minutes before being strained and consumed. It can also be used topically as a poultice or infused oil for skin conditions.

Dosage: The appropriate dosage of chickweed can vary depending on factors such as age, health status, and the specific preparation being used. It's important to follow the recommended dosage on the product label or consult with a qualified herbalist or healthcare professional for personalized guidance.

How to Use: Chickweed tea, infusion, or fresh leaves are typically taken orally. It's often used to soothe inflammation, support digestion, and promote overall well-being. Topically, chickweed can be applied to the skin to alleviate itching, irritation, or minor wounds.

Side Effects: Chickweed is generally considered safe for most people when consumed in moderate amounts. However, some individuals may experience allergic reactions or gastrointestinal upset. It may also interact with certain medications or have adverse effects in individuals with certain health conditions. Pregnant or breastfeeding individuals should consult with a healthcare professional before using chickweed supplements. It's important to use chickweed under the guidance of a healthcare professional and to discontinue use if any adverse effects occur.

Cleavers:

Definition: Cleavers, scientifically known as Galium aparine, is a herbaceous annual plant native to Europe, North America, Asia, and Australia. It has a long history of use in traditional medicine for its potential health benefits.

Ingredients: Cleavers contains various bioactive compounds, including iridoid glycosides, flavonoids, tannins, and mucilage. These compounds are believed to contribute to the herb's medicinal properties, including its potential as a diuretic, lymphatic tonic, and mild astringent.

How to Prepare: Cleavers is typically consumed as an herbal tea, infusion, or in fresh salads. To make tea, dried cleavers leaves and stems are steeped in hot water for several minutes before being strained and consumed. It can also be used topically as a poultice or infused oil for skin conditions.

Dosage: The appropriate dosage of cleavers can vary depending on factors such as age, health status, and the specific preparation being used. It's important to follow the recommended dosage on the product label or consult with a qualified herbalist or healthcare professional for personalized guidance.

How to Use: Cleavers tea, infusion, or fresh leaves are typically taken orally. It's often used to support lymphatic drainage, promote urinary tract health, and soothe inflammation. Topically, cleavers can be applied to the skin to alleviate itching, irritation, or minor wounds.

Side Effects: Cleavers is generally considered safe for most people when consumed in moderate amounts. However, some individuals may experience allergic reactions or gastrointestinal upset. It may also interact with certain medications or have adverse effects in individuals with certain health conditions. Pregnant or breastfeeding individuals should consult with a healthcare professional before using cleavers supplements. It's important to use cleavers under the guidance of a healthcare professional and to discontinue use if any adverse effects occur.

Eucalyptus:

Definition: Eucalyptus refers to a genus of flowering trees and shrubs, primarily native to Australia but also found in other parts of the world. Eucalyptus essential oil, extracted from the leaves of certain species, has a long history of use in traditional medicine for its potential health benefits.

Ingredients: Eucalyptus essential oil contains various bioactive compounds, including eucalyptol (cineole), terpenes, and flavonoids. These compounds are believed to contribute to the oil's medicinal properties, including its potential as an expectorant, decongestant, antiseptic, and anti-inflammatory.

How to Prepare: Eucalyptus essential oil can be used in aromatherapy, diffused in the air, or diluted and applied topically to the skin. It can also be added to steam inhalations or chest rubs to help relieve respiratory symptoms.

Dosage: The appropriate dosage of eucalyptus essential oil can vary depending on factors such as age, health status, and the specific application being used. It's important to follow the recommended dosage on the product label or consult with a qualified aromatherapist or healthcare professional for personalized guidance.

How to Use: Eucalyptus essential oil can be used aromatically, topically, or internally, depending on the intended application. It's often used to alleviate respiratory congestion, soothe sore muscles, promote relaxation, and support overall well-being.

Side Effects: Eucalyptus essential oil is generally considered safe for most people when used appropriately. However, it can be toxic if ingested in large amounts and should not be applied directly to the skin without proper dilution. Some individuals may experience allergic reactions or respiratory irritation when exposed to eucalyptus oil. It's important to use eucalyptus oil with caution, especially around children and pets. Pregnant or breastfeeding individuals should consult with a healthcare professional before using eucalyptus oil. If any adverse effects occur, discontinue use and seek medical attention.

Feverfew:

Definition: Feverfew, scientifically known as Tanacetum parthenium, is a perennial herb native to Europe but also found in other parts of the world. It has a long history of use in traditional medicine, particularly in European folk medicine, for its potential health benefits.

Ingredients: Feverfew contains various bioactive compounds, including sesquiterpene lactones (such as parthenolide), flavonoids, and volatile oils. These compounds are believed to contribute to the herb's medicinal properties, including its potential as an anti-inflammatory, analgesic, and migraine prophylactic.

How to Prepare: Feverfew is typically consumed as an herbal tea, tincture, or in supplement form (such as capsules or tablets). To make tea, dried feverfew leaves and flowers are steeped in hot water for several minutes before being strained and consumed.

Dosage: The appropriate dosage of feverfew can vary depending on factors such as age, health status, and the specific preparation being used. It's important to follow the recommended dosage on the product label or consult with a qualified herbalist or healthcare professional for personalized guidance.

How to Use: Feverfew tea, tincture, or supplements are typically taken orally. It's often used to alleviate headaches, including migraines, and to support overall well-being.

Side Effects: Feverfew is generally considered safe for most people when used in moderate amounts. However, some individuals may experience mild side effects such as gastrointestinal upset or allergic reactions. It may also interact with certain medications or have adverse effects in individuals with certain health conditions, such as bleeding disorders or pregnancy. It's important to use feverfew under the guidance of a healthcare professional and to discontinue use if any adverse effects occur.

Ginseng:

Definition: Ginseng refers to several species of perennial plants belonging to the Panax genus, including Panax ginseng (Asian ginseng) and Panax quinquefolius (American ginseng). Ginseng has been used for centuries in traditional medicine, particularly in East Asia, for its potential health benefits.

Ingredients: Ginseng root contains various bioactive compounds, including ginsenosides, polysaccharides, and peptides. These compounds are believed to contribute to the herb's medicinal properties, including its potential as an adaptogen, immune enhancer, and cognitive booster.

How to Prepare: Ginseng is typically consumed as a powdered root, herbal tea, tincture, or in supplement form (such as capsules or tablets). To make tea, dried ginseng root slices are simmered in water for several minutes before being strained and consumed.

Dosage: The appropriate dosage of ginseng can vary depending on factors such as age, health status, and the specific preparation being used. It's important to follow the recommended dosage on the product label or consult with a qualified herbalist or healthcare professional for personalized guidance.

How to Use: Ginseng powder, tea, tincture, or supplements are typically taken orally. It's often used to support energy levels, enhance cognitive function, and promote overall well-being.

Side Effects: Ginseng is generally considered safe for most people when used in moderate amounts. However, some individuals may experience mild side effects such as insomnia, gastrointestinal upset, or headaches. It may also interact with certain medications or have adverse effects in individuals with certain health conditions, such as high blood pressure or diabetes. Pregnant or breastfeeding individuals should consult with a healthcare professional before using ginseng supplements. It's important to use ginseng under the guidance of a healthcare professional and to discontinue use if any adverse effects occur.

Goldenseal:

Definition: Goldenseal, scientifically known as Hydrastis canadensis, is a perennial herb native to North America. It has a long history of use in traditional Native American medicine and later in folk medicine for its potential health benefits.

Ingredients: Goldenseal root contains various bioactive compounds, including alkaloids (such as berberine and hydrastine), flavonoids, and volatile oils. These compounds are believed to contribute to the herb's medicinal properties, including its potential as an antimicrobial, anti-inflammatory, and immune enhancer.

How to Prepare: Goldenseal is typically consumed as an herbal tea, tincture, or in supplement form (such as capsules or tablets). To make tea, dried goldenseal root or leaves are steeped in hot water for several minutes before being strained and consumed.

Dosage: The appropriate dosage of goldenseal can vary depending on factors such as age, health status, and the specific preparation being used. It's important to follow the recommended dosage on the product label or consult with a qualified herbalist or healthcare professional for personalized guidance.

How to Use: Goldenseal tea, tincture, or supplements are typically taken orally. It's often used to support immune function, promote digestive health, and soothe inflammation.

Side Effects: Goldenseal is generally considered safe for most people when used in moderate amounts. However, some individuals may experience mild side effects such as gastrointestinal upset or allergic reactions. It may also interact with certain medications or have adverse effects in individuals with certain health conditions, such as high blood pressure or pregnancy. It's important to use goldenseal under the guidance of a healthcare professional and to discontinue use if any adverse effects occur.

Bio Ferro Tonic:

Definition: Bio Ferro Tonic is a dietary supplement primarily composed of herbs and minerals. It's often marketed as a natural way to support overall health, particularly by promoting blood health and circulation.

Ingredients: Typical ingredients in Bio Ferro Tonic may include a blend of herbs such as burdock root, yellow dock root, sarsaparilla root, and cascara sagrada bark, along with minerals like iron and potassium phosphate.

How to Prepare: Bio Ferro Tonic usually comes in liquid form and is typically taken orally. It's important to follow the instructions on the product label for dosage and administration.

Dosage: The dosage can vary depending on the specific product and individual needs. It's crucial to consult with a healthcare professional or follow the recommended dosage on the product label to avoid potential side effects.

How to Use: Bio Ferro Tonic is often taken by adding the recommended dosage to water or juice and consuming it orally. It's important to shake the bottle well before use and store it according to the manufacturer's instructions.

Side Effects: While Bio Ferro Tonic is generally considered safe when used as directed, some individuals may experience side effects such as digestive discomfort, allergic reactions, or interactions with medications. It's essential to consult with a healthcare provider before starting any new supplement regimen, especially if you have underlying health conditions or are taking medications.

Bladderwrack:

Definition: Bladderwrack is a type of seaweed or marine algae commonly used in traditional medicine and as a dietary supplement. It's known for its potential health benefits, particularly related to thyroid health and weight management.

Ingredients: Bladderwrack contains various nutrients, including iodine, vitamins, minerals, and antioxidants. The primary active components are iodine and fucoidan, a type of carbohydrate found in brown seaweeds.

How to Prepare: Bladderwrack supplements are available in various forms, including capsules, powders, and liquid extracts. They can be taken orally with water or added to smoothies and other beverages.

Dosage: The appropriate dosage of bladderwrack can vary based on factors such as age, health status, and the specific product being used. It's essential to follow the recommended dosage on the product label or consult with a healthcare professional for personalized guidance.

How to Use: Bladderwrack supplements are typically taken orally, either with water or mixed into food or beverages. It's important to follow the instructions on the product label and avoid exceeding the recommended dosage.

Side Effects: While bladderwrack is generally considered safe for most people when used in moderation, excessive intake of iodine from bladderwrack supplements can cause thyroid dysfunction and other adverse effects. Individuals with thyroid disorders, iodine sensitivity, or certain medical conditions should exercise caution and consult with a healthcare provider before using bladderwrack supplements. Common side effects may include digestive upset, allergic reactions, or interactions with medications.

Blood Purifier:

Definition: Blood purifiers are herbal remedies or dietary supplements believed to cleanse or detoxify the blood, often promoting overall health and well-being. They are thought to support the body's natural detoxification processes and improve blood circulation.

Ingredients: Blood purifiers may contain a variety of herbs and botanical extracts known for their purported cleansing and detoxifying properties. Common ingredients include burdock root, red clover, dandelion root, and yellow dock root, among others.

How to Prepare: Blood purifiers are typically available in various forms, including capsules, tablets, powders, and liquid extracts. They are usually taken orally with water or juice, following the recommended dosage on the product label.

Dosage: The dosage of blood purifiers can vary depending on the specific product and individual needs. It's important to adhere to the recommended dosage on the product label or consult with a healthcare professional for personalized guidance.

How to Use: Blood purifiers are typically taken orally, either with water or mixed into beverages. They are often used as part of a detoxification regimen or to support overall health and vitality.

Side Effects: While blood purifiers are generally considered safe for most people when used as directed, some individuals may experience side effects such as digestive discomfort, allergic reactions, or interactions with medications. It's important to consult with a healthcare provider before starting any new supplement regimen, especially if you have underlying health conditions or are taking medications.

Burdock:

Definition: Burdock, scientifically known as Arctium lappa, is a biennial plant native to Europe and Asia but now found worldwide. It's part of the Asteraceae family and has been used for centuries in traditional medicine and culinary practices.

Ingredients: Burdock contains various nutrients, including carbohydrates, fiber, vitamins (such as vitamin B6, folate, and vitamin C), and minerals (including potassium, magnesium, and manganese). It also contains active compounds such as polyphenols and volatile oils.

How to Prepare: Burdock can be prepared and consumed in various ways. The roots, leaves, and seeds are all utilized for different purposes. The root is commonly used in cooking, herbal teas, tinctures, and supplements, while the leaves and seeds are sometimes used in herbal preparations.

Dosage: The appropriate dosage of burdock root can vary depending on the specific form and intended use. For culinary purposes, there are no strict dosage guidelines, but for supplements or herbal remedies, it's essential to follow the recommended dosage on the product label or consult with a healthcare professional.

How to Use: Burdock root can be used in cooking by peeling, slicing, and adding it to soups, stews, stir-fries, or salads. It can also be brewed into a tea or used to make tinctures or extracts for medicinal purposes. Some people may also take burdock root supplements in capsule or powder form.

Side Effects: While burdock is generally considered safe for most people when consumed in moderate amounts, some individuals may experience allergic reactions or digestive upset. Additionally, burdock may interact with certain medications or have adverse effects in individuals with certain health conditions, such as diabetes or allergies to plants in the Asteraceae family. It's important to consult with a healthcare provider before using burdock, especially if you have underlying health conditions or are taking medications.

Cascara Sagrada:

Definition: Cascara Sagrada, scientifically known as Rhamnus purshiana, is a species of buckthorn native to western North America. It has been used traditionally as a laxative and to promote bowel regularity.

Ingredients: The primary active ingredients in cascara sagrada are anthraquinone glycosides, particularly cascarosides A and B. These compounds stimulate peristalsis in the colon, leading to increased bowel movements.

How to Prepare: Cascara sagrada is typically prepared as an herbal tea, tincture, or capsule. To make tea, dried cascara sagrada bark is steeped in hot water for several minutes before being strained and consumed. Tinctures are prepared by steeping the bark in alcohol to extract its active compounds.

Dosage: The appropriate dosage of cascara sagrada can vary depending on the specific preparation and intended use. It's important to follow the recommended dosage on the product label or consult with a healthcare professional for personalized guidance.

How to Use: Cascara sagrada tea or tincture is typically taken orally. It's important to start with a low dose and gradually increase if needed to avoid potential side effects such as cramping or diarrhea.

Side Effects: Cascara sagrada is considered safe for short-term use when used as directed. However, long-term or excessive use may lead to dependence, electrolyte imbalance, or dehydration. It may also interact with certain medications or have adverse effects in individuals with certain health conditions. It's important to use cascara sagrada under the guidance of a healthcare professional and to discontinue use if any adverse effects occur.

Blue Vervain:

Definition: Blue vervain, also known as Verbena hastata, is a perennial herb native to North America. It has been used in traditional medicine for centuries to treat various ailments, including anxiety, insomnia, and digestive issues.

Ingredients: Blue vervain contains several active compounds, including aucubin, verbenalin, and volatile oils. These compounds are believed to contribute to the herb's medicinal properties.

How to Prepare: Blue vervain is typically consumed as a tea or tincture. To make tea, dried blue vervain leaves and flowers are steeped in hot water for several minutes before being strained and consumed. Tinctures are prepared by steeping the herb in alcohol or vinegar to extract its active compounds.

Dosage: The appropriate dosage of blue vervain can vary depending on factors such as age, health status, and the specific preparation being used. It's important to follow the recommended dosage on the product label or consult with a qualified herbalist or healthcare professional for personalized guidance.

How to Use: Blue vervain tea or tincture is typically taken orally. It can be consumed on its own or mixed with honey or other herbal teas for added flavor.

Side Effects: While blue vervain is generally considered safe for most people when used in moderation, excessive intake may cause digestive upset or allergic reactions in some individuals. Pregnant or breastfeeding women should avoid blue vervain due to its potential to stimulate uterine contractions. As with any herbal remedy, it's important to consult with a healthcare provider before using blue vervain, especially if you have underlying health conditions or are taking medications.

Bromide Plus Powder:

Definition: Bromide Plus Powder is a dietary supplement formulated to support thyroid health and promote overall well-being. It typically contains a blend of herbs and minerals that are believed to have beneficial effects on thyroid function.

Ingredients: Bromide Plus Powder often contains a combination of herbs such as bladderwrack, sea moss, and burdock root, along with minerals like iodine and potassium phosphate. These ingredients are thought to support thyroid function and maintain optimal iodine levels in the body.

How to Prepare: Bromide Plus Powder is usually mixed with water or juice to create a drinkable solution. It's important to follow the instructions on the product label for dosage and preparation.

Dosage: The dosage of Bromide Plus Powder can vary depending on the specific product and individual needs. It's crucial to consult with a healthcare professional or follow the recommended dosage on the product label to avoid potential side effects.

How to Use: Bromide Plus Powder is typically taken orally by mixing the recommended dosage with water or juice. It's important to shake or stir the mixture well before consuming it to ensure even distribution of the ingredients.

Side Effects: While Bromide Plus Powder is generally considered safe when used as directed, some individuals may experience side effects such as digestive discomfort or allergic reactions to certain ingredients. It's essential to consult with a healthcare provider before starting any new supplement regimen, especially if you have underlying health conditions or are taking medications.

Bugleweed:

Definition: Bugleweed, also known as Lycopusvirginicus, is a perennial herb native to North America and Europe. It has been used in traditional medicine to treat various conditions, including hyperthyroidism, anxiety, and insomnia.

Ingredients: Bugleweed contains several active compounds, including lithospermic acid, phenolic acids, and flavonoids. These compounds are believed to contribute to the herb's medicinal properties, particularly its ability to regulate thyroid function.

How to Prepare: Bugleweed is commonly consumed as a tea or tincture. To make tea, dried bugleweed leaves and flowers are steeped in hot water for several minutes before being strained and consumed. Tinctures are prepared by steeping the herb in alcohol or vinegar to extract its active compounds.

Dosage: The appropriate dosage of bugleweed can vary depending on factors such as age, health status, and the specific preparation being used. It's important to follow the recommended dosage on the product label or consult with a qualified herbalist or healthcare professional for personalized guidance.

How to Use: Bugleweed tea or tincture is typically taken orally. It can be consumed on its own or mixed with honey or other herbal teas for added flavor.

Side Effects: While bugleweed is generally considered safe for most people when used in moderation, excessive intake may cause digestive upset or allergic reactions in some individuals.

Pregnant or breastfeeding women should avoid bugleweed due to its potential to stimulate uterine contractions. As with any herbal remedy, it's important to consult with a healthcare provider before using bugleweed, especially if you have underlying health conditions or are taking medications.

Hops:

Definition: Hops, scientifically known as Humulus lupulus, is a perennial climbing vine native to Europe, Asia, and North America. It is primarily known for its use in brewing beer but has also been used historically in traditional medicine for its potential health benefits.

Ingredients: Hops flowers contain various bioactive compounds, including bitter acids (such as humulone and lupulone), essential oils, flavonoids, and polyphenols. These compounds are believed to contribute to the herb's medicinal properties, including its potential as a sedative, relaxant, and digestive aid.

How to Prepare: Hops is typically consumed as an herbal tea, tincture, or in supplement form (such as capsules or tablets). To make tea, dried hops flowers are steeped in hot water for several minutes before being strained and consumed.

Dosage: The appropriate dosage of hops can vary depending on factors such as age, health status, and the specific preparation being used. It's important to follow the recommended dosage on the product label or consult with a qualified herbalist or healthcare professional for personalized guidance.

How to Use: Hops tea, tincture, or supplements are typically taken orally. It's often used to promote relaxation, relieve anxiety, and support sleep.

Side Effects: Hops is generally considered safe for most people when used in moderate amounts. However, some individuals may experience mild side effects such as drowsiness, gastrointestinal upset, or allergic reactions. It may also interact with certain medications or have adverse effects in individuals with certain health conditions, such as depression or hormone-sensitive conditions. It's important to use hops under the guidance of a healthcare professional and to discontinue use if any adverse effects occur.

Kelp:

Definition: Kelp refers to several species of large brown algae belonging to the Laminariales order. It is commonly found in underwater forests along rocky coastlines around the world. Kelp has been used for centuries in various cultures, particularly in East Asia, for its nutritional and medicinal properties.

Ingredients: Kelp is rich in various nutrients, including iodine, vitamins (such as vitamin K, vitamin C, and B vitamins), minerals (including calcium, magnesium, and potassium), antioxidants, and fiber. These nutrients are believed to contribute to the seaweed's potential health benefits, including its role in thyroid function, bone health, and immune support.

How to Prepare: Kelp is typically consumed dried, powdered, or in supplement form (such as capsules or tablets). It can also be used in cooking, particularly in soups, salads, and stir-fries. Kelp supplements are available in various forms, including powdered extracts, tablets, and liquid extracts.

Dosage: The appropriate dosage of kelp can vary depending on factors such as age, health status, and the specific preparation being used. It's important to follow the recommended dosage on the product label or consult with a qualified healthcare professional for personalized guidance.

How to Use: Kelp supplements are typically taken orally with water. They can be consumed as part of a daily nutritional regimen to support overall health and well-being. Kelp can also be incorporated into recipes as a flavorful and nutritious ingredient.

Side Effects: While kelp is generally considered safe for most people when consumed in moderate amounts, excessive intake of iodine-rich foods or supplements, including kelp, can lead to thyroid dysfunction or iodine toxicity. Some individuals may also be allergic to seaweed and experience allergic reactions. Pregnant or breastfeeding individuals should consult with a healthcare professional before using kelp supplements. It's important to use kelp under the guidance of a healthcare professional and to discontinue use if any adverse effects occur.

Blessed Thistle:

Definition: Blessed thistle, scientifically known as Cnicusbenedictus, is an annual or biennial herb native to the Mediterranean region but also found in other parts of Europe, Asia, and North Africa. It has been used historically in traditional medicine for its potential health benefits, particularly for digestive and liver health.

Ingredients: Blessed thistle contains various bioactive compounds, including sesquiterpene lactones (such as cnicin), flavonoids, tannins, and essential oils. These compounds are believed to contribute to the herb's medicinal properties, including its potential as a digestive tonic, appetite stimulant, and liver tonic.

How to Prepare: Blessed thistle is typically consumed as an herbal tea, tincture, or in supplement form (such as capsules or tablets). To make tea, dried blessed thistle leaves and flowers are steeped in hot water for several minutes before being strained and consumed.

Dosage: The appropriate dosage of blessed thistle can vary depending on factors such as age, health status, and the specific preparation being used. It's important to follow the recommended dosage on the product label or consult with a qualified herbalist or healthcare professional for personalized guidance.

How to Use: Blessed thistle tea, tincture, or supplements are typically taken orally. It's often used to support digestion, stimulate appetite, and promote liver health.

Side Effects: Blessed thistle is generally considered safe for most people when used in moderate amounts. However, some individuals may experience mild side effects such as gastrointestinal upset or allergic reactions. It may also interact with certain medications or have adverse effects in individuals with certain health conditions, such as hormone-sensitive conditions or bleeding disorders. Pregnant or breastfeeding individuals should consult with a healthcare professional before using blessed thistle supplements. It's important to use blessed thistle under the guidance of a healthcare professional and to discontinue use if any adverse effects occur.

THE END

9 798325 720451